Alexander Trenton

# ANXIETY DISORDERS, ANXIETY ATTACKS AND VAPING

*The Health Risks and How to Quit*

# Contents



1.

    1.

2.

    1.

3.

    1.

4.
	1.
5.
	1.
6.
	1.
7.
	1.
8.
	1.
9.

# 1

# Chapter 1

## What is anxiety?

Anxiety is a normal reaction to danger, the body's automatic fight-or-flight response that is triggered when you feel threatened, under pressure, or are facing a challenging situation, such as a job interview, exam, or first date. In moderation, anxiety isn't necessarily a bad thing. It can help you to stay alert and focused, spur you to action, and motivate you to solve problems. But when anxiety is constant or overwhelming—when worries and fears interfere with your relationships and daily life—you've likely crossed the line from normal anxiety into the territory of an anxiety disorder.

Since anxiety disorders are a group of related conditions rather than a single disorder, symptoms may vary from person to person. One individual may suffer from intense anxiety attacks that strike without warning, while another gets panicky at the thought of mingling at a party. Someone else may struggle with a disabling fear of driving, or uncontrollable, intrusive thoughts. Yet another may live in a constant state of tension, worrying about anything and everything. But despite their different forms, all anxiety disorders illicit an intense fear or worry out of proportion to the situation at hand.

While having an anxiety disorder can be disabling, preventing you from living the life you want, it's important to know that you're not alone. Anxiety disorders are among the most common mental health issues—and are highly treatable. Once you understand your anxiety disorder, there are steps you can take to reduce the symptoms and regain control of your life.

# 2

# Chapter 2

## What is high-functioning anxiety?

"High-functioning anxiety" is a term you may have come across online. It's not a clinical diagnosis but is sometimes used to describe a person who manages to cope with the demands of daily life despite having anxiety. Outwardly, they may seem unflappable. But beneath their calm demeanor, they're plagued by anxious and negative thoughts.

If you have high-functioning anxiety, you might seem proactive, outgoing, organized, and achievement-oriented. You may even come off as a perfectionist or model student or employee. However, your underlying anxiety can still have health consequences, including irritability, insomnia, and muscle tension.

Different people experience anxiety symptoms in different ways. It's important to remember that some people are dealing with struggles that aren't always apparent.

Do I have an anxiety disorder?

If you identify with any of the following seven signs and symptoms, and they just won't go away, you may be suffering from an anxiety disorder:

1. Are you constantly tense, worried, or on edge?
2. Does your anxiety interfere with your work, school, or family responsibilities?
3. Are you plagued by fears that you know are irrational, but can't shake?
4. Do you believe that something bad will happen if certain things aren't done a certain way?
5. Do you avoid everyday situations or activities because they cause you anxiety?
6. Do you experience sudden, unexpected attacks of heart-pounding panic?
7. Do you feel like danger and catastrophe are around every corner?

Signs and symptoms of anxiety disorders

In addition to the primary symptom of excessive and irrational fear and worry, other common emotional symptoms include:

Feelings of apprehension or dread.

Watching for signs of danger.

Anticipating the worst.

Trouble concentrating.

Feeling tense and jumpy.

Irritability.

Feeling like your mind's gone blank.

But anxiety is more than just a feeling. As a product of the body's fight-or-flight response, it also involves a wide range of physical symptoms, including:


- Pounding heart.
- Sweating.
- Headaches.
- Stomach upset.
- Dizziness.
- Frequent urination or diarrhea.
- Shortness of breath.
- Muscle tension or twitches.
- Shaking or trembling.
- Insomnia.
- Because of these physical symptoms, anxiety sufferers often mistake their disorder for a medical illness. They may visit many doctors and make numerous trips to the hospital before their anxiety disorder is finally recognized.

# 3

# Chapter 3

## What is an anxiety attack?

Anxiety attacks, also known as panic attacks, are episodes of intense panic or fear. They usually occur suddenly and without warning. Sometimes there's an obvious trigger—getting stuck in an elevator, for example, or thinking about the big speech you have to give—but in other cases, the attacks come out of the blue.

Anxiety attacks usually peak within 10 minutes, and they rarely last more than 30 minutes. But during that short time, you may experience terror so severe that you feel as if you're about to die or totally lose control. The physical symptoms are themselves so frightening that many people think they're having a heart attack. After an anxiety attack is over, you may worry about having another one, particularly in a public place where help isn't available or you can't easily escape.

Anxiety attack symptoms include:
Surge of overwhelming panic.
Feeling of losing control or going crazy.

Heart palpitations or chest pain.

Feeling like you're going to pass out.

Trouble breathing or choking sensation.

Hyperventilation.

Hot flashes or chills.

Trembling or shaking.

Nausea or stomach cramps.

Feeling detached or unreal.

It's important to seek help if you're starting to avoid certain situations because you're afraid of having a panic attack. The truth is that panic attacks are highly treatable. In fact, many people are panic free within just 5 to 8 treatment sessions.

# 4

# Chapter 4

## Types of anxiety disorders and their symptoms

Anxiety disorders and closely related conditions include:

Generalized anxiety disorder (GAD)

If constant worries and fears distract you from your day-to-day activities, or you're troubled by a persistent feeling that something bad is going to happen, you may be suffering from generalized anxiety disorder (GAD). People with GAD are chronic worrywarts who feel anxious nearly all of the time, though they may not even know why. GAD often manifests in physical symptoms like insomnia, stomach upset, restlessness, and fatigue.

Panic attacks and panic disorder

Panic disorder is characterized by repeated, unexpected panic attacks, as well as fear of experiencing another episode. Agoraphobia, the fear of being somewhere where escape or help would be difficult in the event of a panic attack, may also accompany a panic disorder. If you have agoraphobia, you are likely to avoid public places such as shopping malls, or confined spaces such as an airplane.

## Obsessive-compulsive disorder (OCD)

Obsessive-compulsive disorder (OCD) is characterized by unwanted thoughts or behaviors that seem impossible to stop or control. If you have OCD, you may feel troubled by obsessions, such as a recurring worry that you forgot to turn off the oven or that you might hurt someone. You may also suffer from uncontrollable compulsions, such as washing your hands over and over.

## Hoarding disorder

Hoarding disorder is a chronic difficulty discarding possessions, accompanied by a dysfunctional attachment to even worthless items. It can lead to excessive accumulation of possessions (or animals) and a cluttered living space. You may attribute emotion to inanimate objects, have a strong sentimental attachment to items, or see the use in any object. These beliefs can make discarding items overwhelm you with feelings of anxiety, guilt, or sadness.

## Phobias and irrational fears

A phobia is an unrealistic or exaggerated fear of a specific object, activity, or situation that in reality presents little to no danger. Common phobias include fear of animals (such as snakes and spiders), fear of flying, and fear of needles. In the case of a severe phobia, you might go to extreme lengths to avoid the object of your fear. Unfortunately, avoidance only strengthens the phobia.

Social anxiety disorder

If you have a debilitating fear of being viewed negatively by others and humiliated in public, you may have social anxiety disorder, also known as social phobia. It can be thought of as extreme shyness and in severe cases, social situations are avoided altogether. Performance anxiety (better known as stage fright) is the most common type of social phobia.

Post-traumatic stress disorder (PTSD)

Post-traumatic stress disorder (PTSD) is an extreme anxiety disorder that can occur in the aftermath of a traumatic or life-threatening event. PTSD can be thought of as a panic attack that rarely, if ever, lets up. Symptoms of PTSD include flashbacks or nightmares about the incident, hypervigilance, startling easily, withdrawing from others, and avoiding situations that remind you of the event.

Separation anxiety disorder

While separation anxiety is a normal stage of development, if anxieties intensify or are persistent enough to get in the way of school or other activities, your child may have separation anxiety disorder. They may become agitated at just the thought of being away from mom or dad and complain of sickness to avoid playing with friends or going to school.

Self-help for anxiety

Not everyone who worries a lot has an anxiety disorder. You may feel anxious because of an overly demanding schedule, lack of exercise or sleep, pressure at home or work, or even from too much caffeine. The bottom line is that if your lifestyle is unhealthy and stressful, you're more likely to feel anxious—whether or not you actually have an anxiety disorder.

These tips can help to lower anxiety and manage symptoms of a disorder:

Connect with others. Loneliness and isolation can trigger or worsen anxiety, while talking about your worries face to face can often make them seem less overwhelming. Make it a point to regularly meet up with friends, join a self-help or support group, or share your worries and concerns with a trusted loved one. If you don't have anyone you can reach out to, it's never too late to build new friendships and a support network.

Manage stress. If your stress levels are through the roof, stress management can help. Look at your responsibilities and see if there are any you can give up, turn down, or delegate to others.

Practice relaxation techniques. When practiced regularly relaxation techniques such as mindfulness meditation, progressive muscle relaxation, and deep breathing can reduce anxiety symptoms and increase feelings of relaxation and emotional well-being.

Exercise regularly. Exercise is a natural stress buster and anxiety reliever. To achieve the maximum benefit, aim for at least 30 minutes of aerobic exercise on most days (broken up into short periods if that's easier). Rhythmic activities that require moving both your arms and legs are especially effective. Try walking, running, swimming, martial arts, or dancing.

Get enough sleep. A lack of sleep can exacerbate anxious thoughts and feelings, so try to get seven to nine hours of quality sleep a night.

Be smart about caffeine, alcohol, and nicotine. Caffeine and alcohol can make anxiety worse. And while it may seem like cigarettes are calming, nicotine is actually a powerful stimulant that leads to higher, not lower, levels of anxiety. For help kicking the habit, see How to Quit Smoking.

Put a stop to chronic worrying. Worrying is a mental habit you can learn how to break. Strategies such as creating a worry period, challenging anxious thoughts, and learning to accept uncertainty can significantly reduce worry and calm your anxious thoughts.

# 5

# Chapter 5

## When to seek professional help

While self-help coping strategies can be very effective, if your worries, fears, or anxiety attacks have become so great that they're causing extreme distress or disrupting your daily routine, it's important to seek professional help.

If you're experiencing a lot of physical symptoms, you should start by getting a medical checkup. Your doctor can check to make sure that your anxiety isn't caused by a medical condition, such as a thyroid problem, hypoglycemia, or asthma. Since certain drugs and supplements can cause anxiety, your doctor will also want to know about any prescriptions, over-the-counter medications, herbal remedies, and recreational drugs you're taking.

If your physician rules out a medical cause, the next step is to consult with a therapist who has experience treating anxiety disorders. The therapist will work with you to determine the cause and type of your disorder and devise a course of treatment.

Treatment

Anxiety disorders respond very well to therapy—and often in a relatively short amount of time. The specific treatment approach depends on the type of anxiety disorder and its severity. But in general, most are treated with therapy, medication, or some combination of the two. Cognitive-behavioral therapy and exposure therapy are types of behavioral therapy, meaning they focus on behavior rather than on underlying psychological conflicts or issues from the past. They can help with issues such as panic attacks, generalized anxiety, and phobias.

Cognitive-behavior therapy helps you identify and challenge the negative thinking patterns and irrational beliefs that fuel your anxiety.

Exposure therapy encourages you to confront your fears and anxieties in a safe, controlled environment. Through gradual exposure to the feared object or situation, either in your imagination or in reality, you gain a greater sense of control. As you face your fear without being harmed, your anxiety will diminish.

Medication

If you have anxiety that's severe enough to interfere with your ability to function, medication may help relieve some symptoms. However, anxiety medications can be habit forming and cause unwanted or even dangerous side effects, so be sure to research your options carefully. Many people use anti-anxiety medication when therapy, exercise, or self-help strategies would work just as well or better—minus the side effects and safety concerns. It's important to weigh the benefits and risks of medication so you can make an informed                                         decision.

# 6

# Chapter 6

## Understanding vaping

Vaping involves inhaling the vapor from an e-cigarette, e-pipe, vape pod, vape pen, or similar device. Many kids and teens look at vaping and see a harmless activity. You might think that it's essentially just flavored steam that helps you relax. Or you might believe that vaping is so common among people your own age that the dangers must be overblown.

It's true that vaping is an increasingly common habit among young people. In a 2021 U.S. survey, more than two million middle and high school students said they had used e-cigarettes within the past month. E-cigarettes were far more popular among those students than cigarettes, cigars, and other tobacco products.

Those numbers are alarming to health professionals because the dangers of vaping are very real. The aerosol from vape devices often contains nicotine, an addictive drug that can affect developing brains. On top of that, when you inhale the vapor from your e-cig, you also breathe in a variety of chemicals, some of which may be toxic. So, that seemingly harmless vapor has the potential to adversely affect your physical and mental health.

If you just vape on occasion, learning more about the risks may be enough to convince you to avoid e-cigs in the future. If you're already a habitual vape user, you might find that cutting nicotine out is a difficult process. Maybe you want to quit, but withdrawal symptoms keep steering you back to your vape. Perhaps you're fearful of the health risks of vaping but uncertain how you'll cope without the nicotine. Know that it can be done. With the right information, support, and strategies, you can drop the habit for good and protect your overall health and well-being.

The health effects of vaping

E-cigarettes have been touted as a safer alternative to traditional cigarettes. Some people even switch to vaping to minimize the risks associated with smoking. It's true that vaped aerosols contain fewer toxic chemicals than the smoke from cigarettes. But that doesn't mean vaping is a risk-free activity.

According to a CDC study, roughly 99 percent of e-cigarettes sold in the U.S. have some level of nicotine, and the content isn't always disclosed. Nicotine is a stimulant that raises your heart rate and gives you a temporary high. You might use it to unwind after a long day at school or calm your nerves before going to a big event.

Although many people initially use nicotine to find relief from anxiety or depression, they quickly discover that addiction can develop. And that addiction worsens mental health in the long run.

If you have a nicotine dependency and go too long without the drug, you may begin to feel depressed, anxious, unfocused, or irritable. So, you vape again to reduce those symptoms, and the cycle repeats. This can lead to a distressing situation as you start to feel as if the nicotine addiction holds power over you.

Nicotine can also affect your brain, which continues to develop until you reach your mid-20s. Nicotine interferes with brain development by impairing regions of the brain responsible for learning, focus, mood, and impulse control. This can have consequences for everything from your schoolwork to your social life.

Difficulty retaining information in class or staying focused on your homework could lead to academic challenges. Mood swings and impulsive behavior might lead you to lash out at your closest friends, causing rifts in your social circle.

Toxic chemicals in e-cigarettes

Aside from nicotine, the aerosol from your vape may expose you to other unhealthy chemicals. Formaldehyde, an irritant and probable carcinogen, can form when the liquid is heated. Chemicals like acrolein, diacetyl, and diethylene glycol can damage your lungs. Vaping can also expose your body to metals, such as tin, lead, nickel, and cadmium.

Vaping may pose dangers that researchers have yet to uncover. As recently as 2019, a synthetic form of vitamin E was identified as a possible culprit behind an outbreak of lung injuries among vape users. In addition, one 2021 study of vaping aerosols and liquids identified the presence of nearly 2,000 unknown chemicals.

# 7

# Chapter 7

## Risk of diseases

More and more studies indicate that vaping can affect oral health. Nicotine interferes with blood flow in the gums, and e-cigarette aerosol alters the state of oral bacteria. This raises the risk of periodontal disease, which comes with symptoms such as bad breath, swollen and bleeding gums, difficulty chewing, and loose teeth.

New research also shows that e-cigarette users may have an increased risk of prediabetes and lung diseases, such as asthma and chronic obstructive pulmonary disease (COPD). If you use both e-cigarettes and traditional cigarettes, you further increase your health risks. One study found that people who use both types of nicotine sources significantly raise their odds of cardiovascular disease.

8

# Chapter 8

## How to quit vaping

There are many reasons to stop vaping, but breaking the habit can be a frustrating process. Maybe you manage to avoid e-cigs for a day before giving in to the desire to vape. Then, a sense of shame and regret accompanies the nicotine high. After repeatedly failing to quit, you might feel helpless, discouraged, and begin to wonder if there's something wrong with you.

Know that you're not alone. Nicotine addiction is an issue that many people struggle with. However, a thoughtful and strategic approach to tackling the addiction and related habits can make all the difference.

Start by reflecting on your own motivations for quitting. For most people, quitting e-cigarettes comes with multiple benefits. Write down all of your motivations. Perhaps you want to save money for an important event, but you keep spending money on vape accessories. Or maybe you want to quit vaping to avoid the physical and mental consequences of addiction. If your relationships with friends, partners, or parents have suffered due to your habit, quitting might improve your social life. This list of reasons to quit vaping will help keep you on track when you're tempted to resume the habit.

Next, set a quit date. When do you plan to be completely free of the vaping habit? Pick a day that falls within the next two weeks, so the drive to quit remains strong. However, don't pick a day that you know will be extremely stressful, such as the day of an important test. Once you have your target goal set, you can begin to adjust your behavior and break the addiction.

Quitting vaping tip 1: Identify and manage triggers

Triggers are specific situations that increase your urge to vape. For example, smelling vapor in the air or seeing friends vape might increase your craving. Maybe online or television ads tempt you to pick up an e-cigarette.

Certain emotional states can also act as triggers. Perhaps the stress of prepping for a job interview increases your desire to vape. You might also turn to nicotine to cope with loneliness and boredom.

If you have a hard time identifying your triggers, keep a craving journal. Record information such as when the craving started, what you were doing, and who you were with. You can also note the intensity of the craving.

Overcoming triggers

Once you know your triggers, you can develop strategies to avoid or minimize them.

For starters, take time to get rid of any vape accessories in your backpack, locker, car, or room. If social pressure is a trigger, take a break from friends who vape or let them know you're trying to quit. If someone tries to coerce you into using e-cigs again, simply give a firm but polite "no thank you." A good friend will respect that boundary.

When it comes to emotion-based triggers, you'll need to learn new ways to cope with those emotions. Here are just a few examples of potential coping strategies:

If you're experiencing loneliness and boredom:

- Use self-compassion and positive self-talk to challenge shyness and anxiety.
- Join clubs and attend events that match your interests.
- Look for opportunities to do volunteer work.

If you're stressed or anxious:

- Incorporate daily mindfulness meditation or breathing exercises.
- Avoid overcommitting and taking on too much responsibility.

- Take care of your body by getting enough sleep and eating a healthy diet.

If you're feeling depressed:

- Use regular physical activity to improve your mood.
- Surround yourself with friends and family members who make you feel safe and cared for.
- Reach out to a helpline if you feel overwhelmed by negative thoughts.

Tip 2: Prepare for cravings and withdrawal

Nicotine withdrawal symptoms are uncomfortable sensations that set in shortly after you quit vaping. They might last days or weeks but know that they're a normal part of the process. Common nicotine withdrawal symptoms can include:

- Cravings
- Irritability
- Grogginess and difficulty concentrating
- Anxiousness
- Restlessness
- Headaches
- Hunger
- Insomnia

Cravings can be intense, but they usually only last for a few minutes. There are plenty of ways to cope until they pass. Experiment with these strategies to see what works best for you.

Have go-to distractions. These could include listening to music, playing with a pet, or playing a video game.

Get physically active. Take a short jog, ride your bike, or do some push-ups or jumping jacks. These activities can serve as distractions, but they can also boost your mood and energize you.

Review your reasons for quitting. Remember that list of your motivations to quit? Revisit it. Reflect on how much better you'll feel once you drop the habit. Envision yourself being free of nicotine.

Use an oral substitute for vaping. For example, chewing gum or crunching on a carrot can help distract you.

Practice deep breathing to calm your nervous system. Slowly inhale through your nose for several seconds. Follow this with a longer exhale. Repeat until you feel your anxiety decrease—or try our Deep Breathing Meditation.

Drink more water. If the cravings come with other withdrawal symptoms, such as headaches and hunger, staying hydrated can help.

Although cravings are common in the first few days of quitting, you'll likely find that they eventually decrease in both frequency and intensity.

Tip 3: Find support

Dropping the habit is ultimately your own responsibility, but leaning on others for support can help. Tell your loved ones that you're trying to quit vaping and would like their backing. Talking to them about your goal will also help them understand any changes in your mood over the next few days or weeks.

Let them know what specific actions they can take to help you. Maybe you want friends to avoid vaping around you. Perhaps you want your brother to bluntly remind you of the health consequences. You might want a friend to join you in a new exercise routine or hobby to reduce your stress and boredom. Remember to take the time to show your appreciation for supportive friends and family members.

You can also look for professional support. Reach out to a cessation counselor for personalized advice on quitting. You can contact a counselor by phone or online. Your doctor might be able to prescribe medication that eases withdrawal symptoms, if necessary. However, you can also find over-the-counter solutions, such as gum and patches.

Be patient with yourself. It might seem difficult at first, but with effort you can kick the habit. Of course, quitting is no small task. So, as you reach each milestone, take time to celebrate your accomplishments. If you slip up and cave to the temptation to vape, don't be too hard on yourself. Turn it into a learning experience. What triggered you to vape again? What can you do to address that trigger in the future?

Tips for parents of children who vape

If your child vapes, it's natural to feel worried. You might fear that vaping will have serious health consequences or lead them to adopt other risky habits.

Despite your fears, you also know that talking to teens about these kinds of subjects can be tricky. You may not want to run the risk of an argument or make them feel defensive. Fortunately, there are many ways to gracefully broach the subject.

First, it's helpful to understand why your child or teen is vaping to start with.

Why kids and teens vape

The more you understand the reasons why young people vape, the easier it will be to talk to your child about the dangers. Common reasons include:

Peer pressure. Many kids and teens say they initially tried e-cigarettes because their friends were using them. Friends might pressure one another to vape by downplaying the risks. Even when there's no overt pressure from friends, non-vaping teens might feel the need to try it out to fit in with the group.

Attractive flavors. Although vape manufacturers avoid directly advertising to younger users, kids and teens often find flavored products appealing. Products that mimic the taste of fruit, candy, and desserts can be particularly enticing.

Negative emotions. Adolescence can be a turbulent time that's filled with self-discovery, social stressors, and school demands. Young e-cigarette users often rely on their vape devices to manage the stress, anxiety, and depression that come with this stage of life.

Perception of safety. For years, e-cigarettes have successfully been pitched as safer alternatives to traditional cigarettes. Unfortunately, kids and teens have also picked up on this messaging and often underestimate the risks of vaping. The sweet flavors can also play into the harmless appearance of vape products.

Accessibility. It's often easier for young people to obtain e-cigarettes, especially if the products are popular among their friend groups. Vaping is also often cheaper than other tobacco products, which is appealing to young people who don't have income.

Aesthetics. Many vape devices are easy to conceal from adults but have a sleek design that teens can show off to one another. Some young people may also think that vaping makes them look older and more mature.

How to talk to your child about vaping

Setting the right tone can make a big difference in how well the conversation goes. You don't need to make the conversation seem like a big deal by pulling your child into the dining room for a formal chat. In fact, this might make them feel interrogated.

Take a casual approach and let the topic come up naturally. For example, maybe you both see an ad on TV or spot someone vaping in public. Situations like those offer a great opportunity to raise the subject. Avoid starting the conversation when you or your child are already stressed or in a rush. The chat might go more smoothly if you're both comfortable.

Use open-ended questions to invite discussion. You can try asking what their opinion is on vaping or the risks of e-cigarettes versus cigarettes. The goal is to have a conversation rather than a lecture. Don't criticize them. Listen to their answers in a nonjudgmental way and ask follow-up questions.

Share what you know about the risks of vaping. You might want to mention how vaping affects the teeth and gums, as well as the potential for nicotine addiction. You can also mention the illegality of underage vaping, but avoid making threats. Make it clear that your concerns come from a place of love rather than the desire to control their every action.

The conversation doesn't need to be one, long chat. You can have many short talks with your child over the span of days, weeks, or months. If your child is initially hesitant to open up about their experiences, return to the topic later. Thinking of it as an ongoing conversation also gives you both time to research and learn more between discussions.

# 9

# Chapter 9

## How to help your child quit vaping

Your support can make all the difference in helping your child kick their vaping habit. Start by educating yourself on addiction and withdrawal symptoms. The more you know about these subjects, the better prepared you'll be to help your child quit.

Help them cope with triggers and temptations. Sit down with your child and make a list of potential triggers. Then, you can work together to brainstorm coping strategies, such as:

- Getting rid of vape devices.
- Practicing saying "no" to peer pressure.
- Keeping gum or other smoking substitutes on hand.

Regularly talk with your child about their stressors. Do they feel depressed about a breakup or anxious about an upcoming test? You don't always need to have solutions to their problems or nuggets of parental wisdom. Sometimes just listening and making your child feel heard is enough to improve their well-being.

Encourage your child to embrace hobbies and social activities. Suggest that they try out team sports, learn an instrument, or join a local club that matches their interests. If they have existing hobbies, do what you can to support them. As your child focuses more on their hobbies and interests, they may feel less tempted to use vaping to manage negative emotions. Volunteer opportunities can also alleviate boredom, boost self-esteem, and help foster a sense of direction.

Make them feel empowered. Compliment their ability to think critically and independently. Let them know you trust them to make smart decisions, even in the face of peer pressure. Remind them of other hurdles they've overcome and things they've accomplished when they put their mind to it. By doing this, you help your child tap into the self-confidence and emotional resilience they need to overcome addiction and quit vaping.